D1104615

The Klinio Diet Solution

Defeat Diabetes and Reclaim Your Health

Nourish Bloomfield

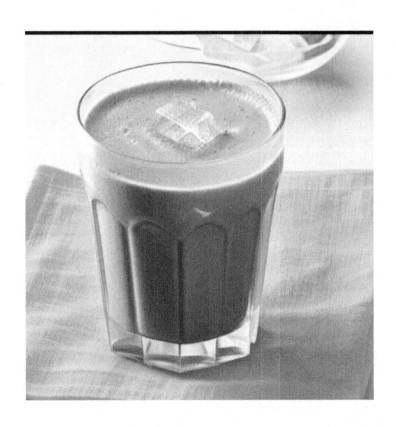

All rights reserved. No part of this publication may be reproduced, distributed, or transmitted in any form or by any means, including photocopying, recording, or other electronic or mechanical methods, without the prior written permission of the publisher, except in the case of brief quotations embodied in critical reviews and certain other noncommercial uses permitted by copyright law.

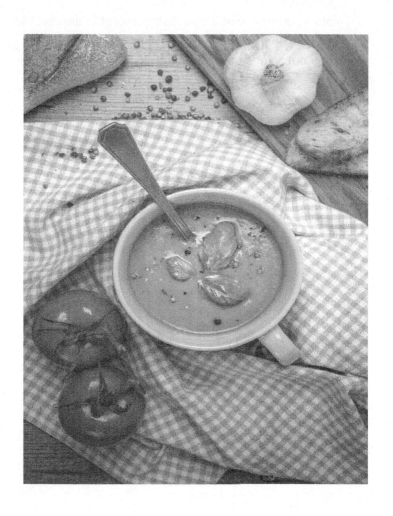

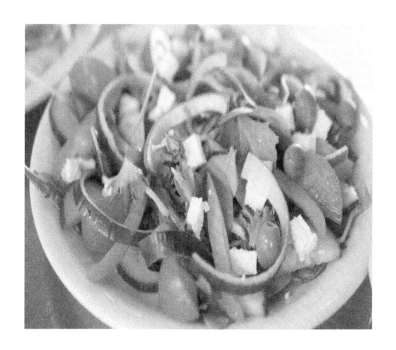

Table Of Contents

Introducing the Klinio Diet: A Life-Changing Journey to Conquering Diabetes

Are you ready to take charge of your health and overcome the challenges of chronic diabetes? Well, buckle up because I'm about to share an incredible success story that will leave you feeling inspired and ready to transform your life.

Imagine a world where you're no longer a prisoner to your condition, where you have the power to manage your blood sugar levels and reclaim your vitality. This is the world that Sarah Werner, a true champion, discovered through the Klinio Diet.

Sarah's journey began with a diagnosis of type 2 diabetes at the age of 28. It hit her hard, shaking her sense of normalcy. Suddenly, her daily routine revolved around insulin shots and constant vigilance over her diet. She tried countless diets, hoping for a breakthrough, but nothing seemed to work. Frustration and exhaustion were her constant companions, and she wondered if she would ever find the key to a better life.

But then, like a beacon of hope, the Klinio Diet entered Sarah's life. It's not just another fad or a quick fix; it's a scientifically grounded meal plan designed specifically for people with diabetes. The Klinio Diet empowers individuals to manage their blood sugar levels, shed excess weight, and embrace a vibrant, fulfilling life.

With nothing to lose and everything to gain, Sarah embarked on her Klinio Diet journey. The results were nothing short of astounding. Within days, her blood sugar levels stabilized, offering her a newfound sense of control. As the pounds began to melt away, her energy skyrocketed, and she experienced a zest for life she thought she had lost forever.

Sarah's transformation is a testament to the power of the Klinio Diet. It's more than just a diet; it's a life-altering approach backed by clinical evidence. The Klinio Diet is built upon a foundation of whole, unprocessed foods and emphasizes low-carb, high-fiber choices that keep blood sugar levels in check. It embraces the importance of healthy fats, which can enhance insulin sensitivity and pave the way for sustainable weight loss.

Now, Sarah is a warrior, a voice of inspiration for the diabetes community. She believes so strongly in the Klinio Diet that she urges everyone with diabetes to give it a chance. She knows firsthand the profound impact it can have on your well-being and quality of life.

So, my friend, if you find yourself wrestling with the challenges of diabetes, I implore you to explore the pages of this book. Let it be your guide on this life-changing journey. Discover a world where delicious meals and vibrant health are intertwined, where you hold the key to unlocking your full potential.

Don't let diabetes define you. Embrace the power of the Klinio Diet and take control of your destiny. The choice is yours, and it could be the most pivotal decision you'll ever make.

Are you ready to embark on this empowering adventure? If so, open this book and let the Klinio Diet be your guiding light to a future free from the shackles of diabetes. Your journey begins now.

Recipes

There is no one-size-fits-all recipe that can cure or fight diabetes. However, there are some general principles that can help people with diabetes make healthy breakfast choices.

- Choose foods that are high in fiber and protein. Fiber and protein can help to slow down the absorption of carbohydrates into the bloodstream, which can help to prevent blood sugar spikes. Good sources of fiber and protein include: Whole grains, such as oatmeal, whole-wheat bread, and quinoa, Eggs, Yogurt, Nuts and seeds

- Avoid sugary foods and drinks. Sugary foods and drinks can quickly raise blood sugar levels. Good alternatives to sugary breakfast foods and drinks include: Fruit, Plain yogurt with berries, Unsweetened almond milk or soy milk, Coffee or tea with no sugar or milk

- Make sure to eat breakfast every day. Skipping breakfast can lead to high blood sugar levels later in the day.

Here are some specific recipes that can help people with diabetes manage their weight and blood sugar levels:

Breakfast

Oatmeal with berries and nuts:

Oatmeal is a good source of fiber, and berries and nuts are a good source of protein. This breakfast is a filling and healthy way to start the day.

Prep Time: 10 minutes
Servings: 1

Ingredients:
- 1/2 cup rolled oats
- 1 cup water
- 1/2 teaspoon cinnamon
- 1/4 teaspoon vanilla extract
- 1/4 cup mixed berries (such as blueberries, raspberries, or strawberries)
- 1 tablespoon chopped nuts (such as almonds, walnuts, or pecans)
- 1 teaspoon chia seeds (optional)
- 1 teaspoon honey

Preparation:
1. In a small saucepan, combine the rolled oats, water, cinnamon, and vanilla extract. Bring the mixture to a boil over medium heat.
2. Reduce the heat to low and simmer for about 5 minutes, stirring occasionally, until the oats are cooked and have absorbed most of the water.
3. Remove the saucepan from the heat and let the oatmeal sit for a minute to thicken.
4. Transfer the oatmeal to a serving bowl.

5. Top the oatmeal with mixed berries, chopped nuts, and chia seeds (if using).
6. Drizzle honey if desired, adjusting the amount to your taste preference.
7. Gently stir the ingredients together to combine.
8. Allow the oatmeal to cool slightly before enjoying.

Greek yogurt with fruit and chia seeds:

This breakfast is beneficial for individuals with diabetes due to its balanced combination of protein, fiber, and healthy fats. The Greek yogurt provides protein and calcium, which can help stabilize blood sugar levels and promote bone health. The fruit adds natural sweetness and dietary fiber, while the chia seeds contribute additional fiber and omega-3 fatty acids, which can aid in blood sugar regulation. The chopped nuts offer healthy fats and added crunch to the meal.

Prep time: 5 minutes
Servings: 1

Ingredients:
- 1 cup plain Greek yogurt
- 1 small apple, diced
- 1/4 cup mixed berries (such as blueberries, raspberries, or strawberries)
- 1 tablespoon chia seeds
- 1 tablespoon chopped nuts (such as almonds, walnuts, or pistachios)
- 1 teaspoon honey

Preparation:
1. In a bowl, add the Greek yogurt as the base of your breakfast.
2. Top the yogurt with the diced apple and mixed berries.
3. Sprinkle the chia seeds and chopped nuts over the fruit.
4. If desired, drizzle the honey or preferred low-calorie sweetener over the top for added sweetness.
5. Mix all the ingredients together gently to combine.
6. Let the mixture sit for a few minutes to allow the chia seeds to absorb some moisture and thicken the yogurt.
7. Enjoy your delicious and diabetes-friendly breakfast!

Egg white omelet with vegetables:

Egg whites are a good source of protein, and vegetables are a good source of vitamins, minerals, and fiber. This breakfast is a quick and easy way to get a healthy start to the day.

Prep Time: 10 minutes
Servings: 1

Ingredients:
- 4 egg whites
- 1/4 cup diced bell peppers (assorted colors)
- 1/4 cup diced onions
- 1/4 cup sliced mushrooms
- 1/4 cup chopped spinach

- 1/2 teaspoon olive oil
- Salt and pepper to taste
- Fresh herbs (such as parsley or basil) for garnish (optional)

Preparation:

1. Heat the olive oil in a non-stick skillet over medium heat.

2. Add the diced onions, bell peppers, and mushrooms to the skillet. Sauté for 3-4 minutes or until the vegetables are slightly softened.

3. Add the chopped spinach to the skillet and cook for an additional 1-2 minutes until wilted. Remove the cooked vegetables from the skillet and set aside.

4. In a mixing bowl, whisk the egg whites until frothy. Season with salt and pepper to taste.

5. Pour the whisked egg whites into the skillet, ensuring that they cover the entire surface evenly. Allow the egg whites to cook undisturbed for a minute or until the edges start to set.

6. Using a spatula, gently lift the edges of the omelet and tilt the skillet to allow the uncooked egg whites to flow underneath. Continue this process around the edges of the omelet until most of the uncooked egg whites have cooked through.

7. Spread the cooked vegetables evenly over one half of the omelet.

8. Carefully fold the other half of the omelet over the vegetables, creating a semi-circle shape. Cook for an additional minute to ensure the omelet is fully set.

9. Slide the omelet onto a plate and garnish with fresh herbs if desired.

Smoothie with protein powder, fruit, and spinach:

Protein powder is a good source of protein, fruit is a good source of vitamins and minerals, and spinach is a good source of fiber. This smoothie is a quick and easy way to get a nutrient-rich breakfast.

Prep Time: 5 minutes
Servings: 1

Ingredients:
- 1 scoop of high-quality protein powder (choose a low-sugar option suitable for your dietary needs)
- 1 cup of mixed berries (such as blueberries, strawberries, or raspberries)
- 1 small ripe banana
- 1 cup fresh spinach leaves
- 1 tablespoon of chia seeds
- 1 cup unsweetened almond milk (or any preferred milk alternative)
- Ice cubes (optional)

- Water (as needed for desired consistency)

Preparation:
1. Gather all the ingredients and ensure they are clean and ready for use.

2. In a blender, add the protein powder, mixed berries, ripe banana, fresh spinach leaves, and chia seeds.

3. Pour in the unsweetened almond milk (or your preferred milk alternative).

4. Optional: If you prefer a colder and thicker smoothie, add a handful of ice cubes to the blender.

5. Blend the ingredients on high speed until you achieve a smooth and creamy consistency. If the mixture is too thick, add a splash of water and blend again until desired consistency is reached.

6. Taste the smoothie and adjust sweetness if necessary. If desired, you can add a small amount of a low-calorie sweetener like stevia or a teaspoon of honey.

7. Once blended to your satisfaction, pour the smoothie into a glass or bottle.

8. If you're on the go, transfer the smoothie to a portable container for convenience.

9. Enjoy your diabetes-fighting smoothie as a nutritious and satisfying breakfast.

Whole-wheat toast with avocado and a hard-boiled egg:

Whole-wheat toast is a good source of fiber, avocado is a good source of healthy fats, and a hard-boiled egg is a good source of protein. This breakfast is a filling and healthy way to start the day.

Prep Time: 15 minutes
Servings: 1

Ingredients:
- 1 slice of whole-wheat bread
- 1/2 ripe avocado
- 1 hard-boiled egg
- 1/2 teaspoon lemon juice
- Salt and pepper to taste
- Optional toppings: sliced cherry tomatoes, sprouts, or a sprinkle of chia seeds

Preparation:
1. Start by boiling the egg. Place the egg in a saucepan and cover it with water. Bring the water to a boil, then reduce the heat to a simmer and cook the egg for about 9-12 minutes for a hard-boiled consistency. Once done, remove the egg from heat, cool it in cold water, and peel off the shell. Set aside.

2. While the egg is cooking, prepare the avocado spread. Cut the ripe avocado in half, remove the pit, and scoop

out the flesh into a small bowl. Add the lemon juice, salt, and pepper to taste. Mash the avocado with a fork until it reaches a desired consistency. Set aside.

3. Toast the slice of whole-wheat bread until it's golden brown and crispy. Place it on a plate.

4. Spread the prepared avocado mixture evenly over the toasted bread.

5. Take the hard-boiled egg and slice it into rounds or halves. Place the egg slices on top of the avocado spread.

6. If desired, you can add additional toppings such as sliced cherry tomatoes, sprouts, or a sprinkle of chia seeds for added nutrition and flavor.

7. Serve the whole-wheat toast with avocado and hard-boiled egg immediately, while it's still warm.

Lunch

Grilled salmon with roasted vegetables: Salmon is a good source of protein and omega-3 fatty acids, which can help to improve insulin sensitivity. Roasted vegetables are a good source of fiber and vitamins, which can also help to regulate blood sugar levels.

Prep Time: 15 minutes
Servings: 2

Ingredients:
- 2 salmon fillets (about 4-6 ounces each)
- 1 tablespoon olive oil
- 1 teaspoon lemon juice
- Salt and pepper to taste
- 1 cup broccoli florets
- 1 cup cauliflower florets
- 1 medium-sized zucchini, sliced
- 1 medium-sized red bell pepper, sliced
- 1 tablespoon olive oil
- ½ teaspoon garlic powder
- ½ teaspoon dried herbs (such as thyme or rosemary)
- Salt and pepper to taste

Preparation:

1. Preheat your grill to medium heat or use a grill pan on the stovetop.

2. In a small bowl, mix together olive oil, lemon juice, salt, and pepper. Brush this mixture evenly over both sides of the salmon fillets.

3. Place the salmon fillets on the preheated grill or grill pan, skin-side down if applicable. Cook for about 4-6 minutes per side, or until the salmon is cooked through and easily flakes with a fork. Remove from heat and set aside.

Lentil soup: Soup is a filling and satisfying meal that can help to keep blood sugar levels stable. Lentil soup is a good option for people with diabetes because it is low in calories and fat, and it is a good source of protein and fiber.

Prep time: 10 minutes
Cook time: 30 minutes
Servings: 4

Ingredients:
- 1 cup dried lentils (green or brown), rinsed and drained
- 1 tablespoon olive oil
- 1 onion, finely chopped
- 2 cloves garlic, minced
- 2 carrots, diced
- 2 celery stalks, diced
- 1 teaspoon ground cumin
- 1 teaspoon ground turmeric
- 1 teaspoon paprika
- 4 cups low-sodium vegetable broth
- 1 can (14 ounces) diced tomatoes (preferably no added sugar)
- Salt and pepper to taste
- Fresh parsley, chopped (for garnish)

Preparation:

1. Heat the olive oil in a large pot or Dutch oven over medium heat.

2. Add the chopped onion and minced garlic to the pot. Sauté for 2-3 minutes until the onion becomes translucent and the garlic is fragrant.

3. Add the diced carrots and celery to the pot. Cook for an additional 3-4 minutes, stirring occasionally, until the vegetables start to soften.

4. Stir in the ground cumin, turmeric, and paprika, ensuring the vegetables are well coated with the spices.

5. Add the rinsed lentils to the pot, followed by the vegetable broth and diced tomatoes. Stir well to combine all the ingredients.

6. Increase the heat to high and bring the mixture to a boil. Once boiling, reduce the heat to low, cover the pot, and let it simmer for about 25-30 minutes or until the lentils are tender.

7. Season with salt and pepper to taste. Adjust the seasoning according to your preference.

8. Remove the pot from the heat. Using an immersion blender, blend a portion of the soup until desired consistency is reached. This step is optional but helps create a thicker texture.

9. Serve the lentil soup hot, garnished with freshly chopped parsley.

Salad with grilled chicken or tofu: Salad is a healthy and refreshing meal that can help to boost your intake of fruits and vegetables. Grilled chicken or tofu adds protein to the salad, which can help to keep you feeling full.

Prep Time: 20 minutes
Servings: 2

Ingredients:
- 8 ounces of boneless, skinless chicken breast or firm tofu
- 6 cups mixed salad greens (spinach, arugula, lettuce)
- 1 medium cucumber, sliced
- 1 cup cherry tomatoes, halved
- 1 small red onion, thinly sliced
- 1 small avocado, sliced
- 2 tablespoons extra virgin olive oil
- 2 tablespoons lemon juice
- 1 teaspoon Dijon mustard
- Salt and pepper to taste
- Optional toppings: chopped nuts (almonds, walnuts), seeds (sunflower, pumpkin), feta cheese (if tolerated), or low-carb dressing

Preparation:
1. Preheat the grill to medium-high heat. If using tofu, press it between paper towels to remove excess moisture, then cut it into slices or cubes.
2. Season the chicken or tofu with salt and pepper.
3. Grill the chicken or tofu for about 4-6 minutes per side, or until cooked through. Remove from the grill and let it rest for a few minutes. Slice the chicken into thin strips if using.
4. In a large salad bowl, combine the mixed greens, cucumber slices, cherry tomatoes, red onion slices, and avocado.
5. In a small bowl, whisk together the extra virgin olive oil, lemon juice, Dijon mustard, salt, and pepper to make the dressing.

6. Pour the dressing over the salad and toss to coat the ingredients evenly.

7. Divide the salad onto two plates.

8. Arrange the grilled chicken or tofu slices on top of each salad.

9. If desired, add optional toppings such as chopped nuts, seeds, or a sprinkle of feta cheese (if tolerated).

10. Serve the salad immediately and enjoy!

Quinoa bowl with black beans, corn, and avocado: Quinoa is a good source of protein and fiber, which can help to regulate blood sugar levels. Black beans and corn are also good sources of fiber, and they add flavor and texture to the bowl. Avocado adds healthy fats and nutrients to the bowl.

Prep time: 15 minutes
Servings: 2

Ingredients:
- 1 cup cooked quinoa
- 1 cup black beans (cooked or canned, drained and rinsed)
- 1 cup cooked corn kernels
- 1 ripe avocado, diced
- 1 small red bell pepper, diced
- 1 small red onion, finely chopped
- 2 tablespoons fresh cilantro, chopped
- Juice of 1 lime
- 1 tablespoon extra-virgin olive oil
- Salt and pepper to taste

Preparation:

1. In a large mixing bowl, combine the cooked quinoa, black beans, corn kernels, diced avocado, red bell pepper, red onion, and chopped cilantro.

2. In a separate small bowl, whisk together the lime juice, extra-virgin olive oil, salt, and pepper to make the dressing.

3. Pour the dressing over the quinoa mixture and toss gently to coat all the ingredients evenly.

4. Adjust the seasoning according to your taste preferences.

5. Divide the quinoa bowl mixture into two serving bowls.

6. You can optionally garnish the bowls with additional cilantro leaves or lime wedges.

7. Serve the quinoa bowl immediately and enjoy!

Hummus wrap with vegetables: Hummus is a good source of protein and fiber, and it is also a good source of healthy fats. Vegetables add flavor and nutrients to the wrap.

Prep Time: 15 minutes
Servings: 2

Ingredients:
- 4 whole wheat tortillas or wraps
- 1 cup homemade or store-bought hummus (preferably low-sodium)
- 1 small cucumber, thinly sliced

- 1 medium bell pepper, thinly sliced
- 1 medium carrot, grated
- 1 small red onion, thinly sliced
- 2 cups mixed salad greens
- Fresh herbs of your choice (such as parsley or cilantro), chopped (optional)
- Salt and pepper to taste

Preparation:
1. Wash and prepare the vegetables. Slice the cucumber, bell pepper, and red onion into thin strips. Grate the carrot. Set aside.
2. Take the whole wheat tortillas or wraps and lay them flat on a clean surface.
3. Spread a generous layer of hummus (approximately ¼ cup) evenly over each tortilla.
4. Divide the sliced cucumber, bell pepper, grated carrot, red onion, and mixed salad greens evenly among the wraps, placing the ingredients in the center of each tortilla.
5. Sprinkle with fresh herbs if desired, and season with salt and pepper to taste.
6. Carefully roll each tortilla tightly, folding in the sides as you go to create a wrap.
7. Slice each wrap diagonally into halves or leave them whole if preferred.
8. Serve the hummus wraps immediately, or if packing them for later, wrap them tightly in foil or plastic wrap to keep them fresh.

Dinner

Grilled salmon with roasted vegetables: Salmon is a good source of protein and omega-3 fatty acids, both of which can help to improve insulin sensitivity. The roasted vegetables add fiber and vitamins to the dish. Certainly! Here's a recipe for grilled salmon with roasted vegetables that incorporates ingredients known for their potential benefits in managing diabetes:

Prep Time: 15 minutes
Cook Time: 25 minutes
Servings: 2

Ingredients:
- 2 salmon fillets (approximately 6 ounces each)
- 2 tablespoons olive oil
- 1 teaspoon lemon zest
- 1 tablespoon lemon juice
- 1 clove garlic, minced
- Salt and pepper to taste
- 2 cups mixed vegetables (such as bell peppers, zucchini, and broccoli), cut into bite-sized pieces
- 1 tablespoon balsamic vinegar
- 1 teaspoon dried herbs (such as thyme or rosemary)
- 1 tablespoon chopped fresh parsley (for garnish)

Preparation:

1. Preheat the oven to 400°F (200°C).

2. In a small bowl, combine 1 tablespoon olive oil, lemon zest, lemon juice, minced garlic, salt, and pepper. Stir well to create a marinade for the salmon.

3. Place the salmon fillets in a shallow dish and pour the marinade over them. Ensure that the fillets are evenly coated. Allow them to marinate for 10 minutes.

4. Meanwhile, prepare the vegetables. In a separate bowl, toss the mixed vegetables with 1 tablespoon olive oil, balsamic vinegar, dried herbs, salt, and pepper until well coated.

5. Line a baking sheet with parchment paper. Arrange the marinated salmon fillets on one half of the baking sheet, leaving space for the vegetables on the other half.

6. Place the baking sheet in the preheated oven and roast for 10 minutes.

7. After 10 minutes, remove the baking sheet from the oven and add the seasoned vegetables to the empty half of the sheet.

8. Return the baking sheet to the oven and continue roasting for an additional 15 minutes, or until the salmon is cooked through and the vegetables are tender and slightly caramelized.

9. Once cooked, carefully remove the salmon and vegetables from the oven.

10. Serve the grilled salmon fillets alongside the roasted vegetables on a plate. Garnish with chopped fresh parsley.

Chicken stir-fry with brown rice: Stir-fries are a quick and easy way to get a healthy and balanced meal. The chicken is a good source of protein, and the vegetables add fiber and vitamins. Brown rice is a complex carbohydrate that will release energy slowly, which can help to prevent blood sugar spikes.

Prep Time: 15 minutes
Servings: 4

Ingredients:
- 2 boneless, skinless chicken breasts, thinly sliced
- 2 tablespoons low-sodium soy sauce
- 1 tablespoon sesame oil
- 1 tablespoon olive oil
- 2 cloves garlic, minced
- 1-inch piece of ginger, grated
- 1 medium onion, thinly sliced
- 1 red bell pepper, thinly sliced
- 1 yellow bell pepper, thinly sliced
- 1 cup broccoli florets
- 1 cup snap peas, ends trimmed
- 1 medium carrot, julienned
- 2 tablespoons low-sodium chicken broth or water
- 2 tablespoons low-sodium oyster sauce
- 1 tablespoon cornstarch (optional, for thickening)
- 4 cups cooked brown rice

- Fresh cilantro or green onions for garnish (optional)

Preparation:
1. In a bowl, marinate the chicken slices with soy sauce for about 10 minutes while you prepare the vegetables.

2. Heat the sesame oil and olive oil in a large skillet or wok over medium-high heat. Add the minced garlic and grated ginger, and sauté for about 1 minute until fragrant.

3. Add the marinated chicken to the skillet and cook until it is no longer pink and cooked through. Remove the chicken from the skillet and set it aside.

4. In the same skillet, add the sliced onion, bell peppers, broccoli florets, snap peas, and julienned carrot. Stir-fry for about 5 minutes until the vegetables are crisp-tender.

5. In a small bowl, mix the low-sodium chicken broth or water with the low-sodium oyster sauce. Pour the sauce over the vegetables and stir to coat evenly.

6. If desired, you can thicken the sauce by mixing the cornstarch with a little water to make a slurry. Add the slurry to the skillet and stir until the sauce thickens slightly.

7. Return the cooked chicken to the skillet and toss everything together to combine.

8. Serve the chicken stir-fry over cooked brown rice. Garnish with fresh cilantro or green onions if desired.

Lentil soup: Lentils are a good source of protein, fiber, and complex carbohydrates. They are also low on the glycemic index, which means they will not cause a sudden spike in blood sugar levels.

Tofu scramble with vegetables: Tofu is a good source of protein and can be a healthy alternative to meat. The vegetables add fiber and vitamins to the dish.

Black bean burgers: Black beans are a good source of protein and fiber. They are also low on the glycemic index, which means they will not cause a sudden spike in blood sugar levels.

Snacks

Greek yogurt with berries and nut: Greek yogurt is a good source of protein and calcium, both of which can help to regulate blood sugar levels. Berries are a good source of fiber and antioxidants, both of which can also help to fight diabetes. Nuts are a good source of healthy fats, which can help to keep you feeling full and satisfied.

Prep Time: 5 minutes
Servings: 1

Ingredients:
- 1 cup plain Greek yogurt
- 1/2 cup mixed berries (such as strawberries, blueberries, and raspberries)
- 1 tablespoon chopped nuts (such as almonds, walnuts, or pecans)
- 1 teaspoon chia seeds
- 1/2 teaspoon cinnamon (optional)
- 1 teaspoon honey or preferred low-calorie sweetener (optional)

Preparation:
1. In a bowl, scoop out 1 cup of plain Greek yogurt.
2. Wash the mixed berries and add them on top of the yogurt.
3. Sprinkle the chopped nuts and chia seeds over the berries.
4. If desired, add a sprinkle of cinnamon for added flavor and potential blood sugar regulation.
5. Drizzle 1 teaspoon of honey or a preferred low-calorie sweetener over the yogurt for sweetness (optional).
6. Mix all the ingredients together gently, ensuring the berries, nuts, and seeds are evenly distributed throughout the yogurt.
7. Serve the Greek yogurt with berries and nuts immediately or refrigerate for a short period to chill before enjoying.

Apple with peanut butter: Apples are a good source of fiber, which can help to slow down the absorption of carbohydrates into the bloodstream. Peanut butter is a good source of protein and healthy fats, both of which can help to keep you feeling full and satisfied.

Servings: 1
Prep time: 5 minutes
Ingredients:

- 1 apple, sliced
- 2 tablespoons peanut butter

Instructions:

1. Spread the peanut butter on the apple slices.
2. Enjoy!

Vegetable sticks with hummus:
Vegetables are a good source of fiber, which can help to slow down the absorption of carbohydrates into the bloodstream. Hummus is a good source of protein and healthy fats, both of which can help to keep you feeling full and satisfied.

Servings: 1

Prep time: 5 minutes

Ingredients:
- 1 carrot, sliced
- 1 celery stalk, sliced
- 1/2 cup hummus

Instructions:

1. Dip the vegetable sticks in the hummus.
2. Enjoy!

Hard-boiled eggs: Hard-boiled eggs are a good source of protein, which can help to keep you feeling full and satisfied. They are also a good source of choline, a nutrient that has been shown to improve insulin sensitivity.

Servings: 1

Prep time: 10 minutes

Cook time: 10 minutes

Ingredients:
 2 eggs

Instructions:

1. Bring a pot of water to a boil.
2. Gently place the eggs in the boiling water.
3. Cook for 10 minutes.
4. Remove the eggs from the water and run them under cold water until they are cool enough to handle.
5. Peel the eggs and enjoy!

5. Oatcakes with almond butter and bananas

Oatcakes are a good source of fiber, which can help to slow down the absorption of carbohydrates into the bloodstream. Almond butter is a good source of protein and healthy fats, both of which can help to keep you feeling full and satisfied. Bananas are a good source of potassium, a mineral that can help to regulate blood sugar levels.

Servings: 1

Prep time: 5 minutes

Ingredients:

- 1 oatcake
- 1 tablespoon almond butter
- 1/2 banana, sliced

Instructions:

1. Spread the almond butter on the oatcake.
2. Top with the banana slices.
3. Enjoy!

These are just a few examples of snacks that can help fight diabetes. There are many other healthy and delicious snacks that you can enjoy. It is important to talk to your doctor or a registered dietitian to create a snack plan that is right for you.

Desserts

Chocolate avocado mousse:

This mousse is made with avocado, which is a good source of healthy fats and fiber. The healthy fats can help to slow down the absorption of sugar into the bloodstream, and the fiber can help to keep you feeling full. The chocolate in this mousse is made with cocoa powder, which is a good source of antioxidants. Antioxidants can help to protect your cells from damage, which can help to improve your overall health.

Servings: 4

Prep time: 10 minutes

Ingredients:
- 1 ripe avocado, mashed
- 1/4 cup unsweetened cocoa powder
- 1/4 cup stevia powder
- 1/4 cup almond milk
- 1/4 teaspoon vanilla extract

Instructions:
1. In a blender, combine the avocado, cocoa powder, stevia powder, almond milk, and vanilla extract.
2. Blend until smooth.
3. Pour the mousse into serving bowls or glasses.
4. Refrigerate for at least 1 hour before serving.

Strawberry chia pudding

Chia seeds are a good source of fiber, which can help to slow down the absorption of sugar into the bloodstream. Strawberries are a good source of antioxidants and fiber. The combination of chia seeds and strawberries makes this pudding a healthy and delicious dessert option for people with diabetes.

Servings: 4

Prep time: 5 minutes

Ingredients:

- 1 cup chia seeds
- 2 cups unsweetened almond milk
- 1/2 cup strawberries, hulled and sliced
- 1/4 teaspoon vanilla extract

Instructions:

1. In a bowl, combine the chia seeds, almond milk, strawberries, and vanilla extract.
2. Stir until well combined.
3. Cover the bowl and refrigerate for at least 4 hours, or overnight.
4. Serve chilled.

Greek yogurt parfait

Greek yogurt is a good source of protein and calcium. Both protein and calcium can help to keep you feeling full and satisfied after eating. The fruit in this parfait adds fiber and antioxidants. The combination of Greek yogurt and fruit makes this a healthy and delicious dessert option for people with diabetes.

Prep Time: 10 minutes
Servings: 1

Ingredients:
- 1/2 cup plain Greek yogurt (low-fat or non-fat)
- 1/4 cup mixed berries (such as strawberries, blueberries, raspberries)
- 1 tablespoon chopped nuts (e.g., almonds, walnuts, or pistachios)
- 1 tablespoon ground flaxseeds
- 1 teaspoon honey or preferred low-calorie sweetener (optional)
- 1/4 teaspoon cinnamon (optional)

Preparation:
1. In a serving glass or bowl, start by adding a layer of 1/4 cup of plain Greek yogurt.
2. Top the yogurt with half of the mixed berries.
3. Sprinkle half of the chopped nuts and half of the ground flaxseeds over the berries.
4. Drizzle half of the honey or sweetener (if using) over the nuts and seeds.
5. Repeat the layering process by adding another 1/4 cup of Greek yogurt, the remaining mixed berries, remaining chopped nuts, remaining ground flaxseeds, and the rest of the honey or sweetener.

6. If desired, sprinkle cinnamon on top for additional flavor and potential blood sugar regulation.

7. Serve immediately and enjoy!

Apple crisp with cinnamon and nuts:

Apples are a good source of fiber and antioxidants. Cinnamon has been shown to help to regulate blood sugar levels. The nuts in this crisp add healthy fats and protein. The combination of apples, cinnamon, and nuts makes this a healthy and delicious dessert option for people with diabetes.

Servings: 6

Prep time: 15 minutes

Cook time: 30 minutes

Ingredients:
- 6 apples, peeled, cored, and sliced
- 1/4 cup unsweetened applesauce
- 1/4 teaspoon cinnamon
- 1/4 cup chopped nuts (any type)

Instructions:

1. Preheat oven to 375 degrees F (190 degrees C).

2. In a bowl, combine the apples, applesauce, cinnamon, and nuts.

3. Pour the apple mixture into a greased baking dish.

4. Bake for 30 minutes, or until the apples are tender and the topping is golden brown.
5. Serve warm or cold.

Frozen Yoghurt Bark

Frozen yogurt is a good source of protein and calcium. It is also lower in sugar than ice cream. The fruit in this bark adds fiber and antioxidants. The combination of frozen yogurt and fruit makes this a healthy and delicious dessert option for people with diabetes.

Servings: 6

Prep time: 10 minutes

Freeze time: 6 hours

Ingredients:

- 1 pint frozen yogurt
- 1/2 cup berries (any type, chopped)
- 1 tablespoon unsweetened granola

Instructions:

1. In a shallow dish, spread out the frozen yogurt.
2. Top with the fruit and granola.
3. Freeze for at least 6 hours, or overnight.

Smoothies

Green Power Smoothie:

Packed with leafy greens and high-fiber ingredients to help regulate blood sugar levels.

Servings: 1

Prep time: 5 minutes

Ingredients:

- 1 cup spinach
- 1 small cucumber
- 1 green apple
- 1 stalk of celery
- ½ lemon (juiced)
- 1 cup unsweetened almond milk
- Ice cubes (optional)

Preparation:

1. Blend all the ingredients until smooth.
2. Add ice cubes if desired and blend again.
3. Serve chilled.

Berry Blast Smoothie:

Rich in antioxidants, fiber, and vitamins from berries, which may help improve insulin sensitivity.

Servings: 1

Prep time: 5 minutes

Ingredients:

- 1 cup mixed berries (strawberries, blueberries, raspberries)
- ½ cup plain Greek yogurt

- 1 tablespoon chia seeds
- 1 cup unsweetened almond milk
- 1 teaspoon honey or preferred low-calorie sweetener (optional)

Preparation:
1. Combine all the ingredients in a blender and blend until smooth.
2. Adjust sweetness if desired.
3. Serve and enjoy.

Cinnamon Banana Smoothie:

Cinnamon has been suggested to have potential blood sugar-lowering effects.
Servings: 1
Prep time: 5 minutes
Ingredients:
- 1 ripe banana
- 1 cup unsweetened almond milk
- ½ teaspoon ground cinnamon
- 1 tablespoon almond butter
- 1 teaspoon honey or preferred low-calorie sweetener (optional)

Preparation:
1. Place all the ingredients in a blender and blend until creamy and well combined.
2. Add sweetener if desired.
3. Pour into a glass and serve.

Avocado Spinach Smoothie:

Avocado provides healthy fats and fiber, which can aid in blood sugar control.

Servings: 1

Prep time: 5 minutes

Ingredients:

- ½ ripe avocado
- 1 cup spinach
- 1 small ripe banana
- 1 cup unsweetened almond milk
- 1 tablespoon almond butter
- Ice cubes (optional)

Preparation:

1. Combine all the ingredients in a blender and blend until smooth.
2. Add ice cubes if desired and blend again.
3. Pour into a glass and enjoy.

Tropical Turmeric Smoothie: Turmeric contains curcumin, which has shown potential anti-inflammatory and blood sugar-lowering effects.

Servings: 1

Prep time: 5 minutes

Ingredients:

- 1 cup frozen pineapple chunks
- 1 small ripe banana
- ½ teaspoon ground turmeric
- 1 tablespoon grated ginger
- 1 cup unsweetened coconut milk
- 1 teaspoon honey or preferred low-calorie sweetener (optional)

Preparation:
1. Place all the ingredients in a blender and blend until smooth.
2. Adjust sweetness if desired.
3. Pour into a glass and serve.

Conclusion

We've reached the end of this incredible journey through the Klinio Diet, and I hope you're feeling as pumped up as I am. Together, we've explored the power of nutrition, the potential to conquer diabetes, and the delicious recipes that fuel our bodies and our souls.

But this is just the beginning. The Klinio Diet isn't just a collection of recipes; it's a gateway to a whole new world of possibilities. It's a reminder that we hold the power to shape our own destinies, no matter the challenges we face.

As you close this book, remember the stories we've shared, the mouthwatering meals we've discovered, and the victories that lie ahead. Take this knowledge and go forth with confidence, armed with the tools to make positive changes in your life.

I want to leave you with this: You have the power to transform your health, to embrace a life full of vitality and joy. The Klinio Diet has given you the foundation, but it's up to you to take action, to make those small changes that will lead to lasting results.

So, my friend, go out there and live your best life. Embrace the flavors, the nourishment, and the passion for living well. Let the Klinio Diet be your compass, guiding you towards a future brimming with energy and fulfillment.

Thank you for joining me on this remarkable journey. I can't wait to hear your success stories and witness the incredible impact the Klinio Diet has on your life. Remember, you have the power within you, and now you have the recipes to make it happen.

Stay hungry for greatness, my friends. The world is yours for the taking.

Signing off,
Nourish Bloomfield

Klinio Diet Journal

Days	Recipes	Remarks
1		
2		
3		
4		
5		
6		
7		
8		
9		
10		
11		
13		
13		
14		

15		
16		
17		
18		
19		

20		
21		
22		
23		
24		
25		
26		
27		
28		
29		
30		

Made in the USA
Coppell, TX
27 August 2023

20867305R00031